Making Milk Soap

excerpted from *Milk-Based Soaps* by Casey Makela

CONTENTS

Introduction

Soapmaking is a blend of science and art. Once you have mastered the technique of mixing fats and alkalis to make soap, you can unleash your imagination. Learn the basics of soapmaking, then experiment with colors, shapes, scents, and textures to create one-of-a-kind handicrafts.

Soap is created when a fat is mixed with an alkali. When the two ingredients combine, a chemical reaction occurs. This reaction is known as *saponification.*

Soap can be made with either animal or vegetable fats. In this bulletin, vegetable fats are used, since they complement the gentle nature of milk-based soaps. The alkali used most often in home-based soapmaking is sodium hydroxide. It's commonly called caustic soda or lye. This bulletin uses the term *lye.*

Milk has long been revered as a cosmetic ingredient. It's an excellent moisturizer and has been heralded throughout the ages as a skin softener that even the most delicate skin types can trust. Milk makes soap richer, creamier, and less drying to the skin.

A Glance Back

Soap is mentioned in the writings of Pliny the Elder, the first-century naturalist and historian. In 77 A.D., Pliny described various forms of hard and soft soaps that were used by women to make their hair shine. An extensive soap factory was discovered among the ruins of Pompeii, an ancient Roman resort. Despite efforts by the Christian church to discourage bathing as immodest, soap was valued as an article of commerce in early Europe.

In the 13th century, Italy introduced soapmaking to France. At that time, most soap was made by boiling goat tallow with beechwood ash and water. French soapmakers refined the quality of soap by using olive oil instead of animal fats. Around 1500, the French introduced soap to England, where the industry grew rapidly.

Soap Comes to America

In the American colonies, soapmaking was as important as spinning, weaving, candlemaking, and other common domestic skills. Fats were rendered from slaughtered livestock. Trees, especially hardwoods, were burned to create a fine ash. The ashes were kept in a leaching barrel — a large wooden barrel with a plugged hole near the base.

A thin layer of stones was placed in the bottom, then the barrel was filled with straw and ashes. Leaching barrels were kept close to the house or barn where they could catch rain runoff. Once the ashes in the leaching barrel were saturated, the plug was removed and enough lye-water for a batch of soap was drained into a non-metal container.

A common test of the lye-water's strength was to dip a feather in it. If the feather dissolved, the lye-water was strong enough to make soap. If not, the water was poured back into the leaching barrel to strengthen. The caustic lye-water could easily burn the skin and the added danger of stirring a kettle filled with hot fats over an open fire made soapmaking hazardous.

In 1621, soap ash was an important and lucrative export from America to England, providing the colonies with a much needed source of income. Settlements in what are now Maine and New Hampshire gained great wealth from soap ash and fat exports to England.

Modern Soapmaking

Using wood ash to produce enough alkali for soapmaking was tedious, time consuming, and labor intensive. In 1791, Nicolas Leblanc discovered a process for inexpensively manufacturing caustic soda on a large scale. Leblanc's discovery revolutionized the soap industry and eliminated the need to import soap from the colonies.

The chemist M.E. Chevreul characterized the differences between fats and oils in the 1800s. His research uncovered the underlying principles of saponification. No discovery has contributed more to the basic, comprehensive understanding of soapmaking than Chevreul's.

Leblanc's and Chevreul's discoveries helped to modernize the soapmaking process. By the first half of the 19th century, large-scale manufacturing operations were in place. It was common for soap to be manufactured in huge kettles containing 100,000 to 1 million pounds of liquid soap. These kettles were heated by open fires and the contents were constantly stirred until the soap was ready to be poured. Then, the mixture was hand-ladled into large wooden molds, where the saponifying soap hardened until it could be cut.

An early American soap manufacturing company was founded in 1806 by William Colgate of New York. By 1850, New England was the principal center of soap manufacturing in the United States. The introduction of perfumed and colored soaps was the beginning of the multibillion-dollar soap industry of today.

Commercial soapmaking barely resembles the simplicity of early production in either ingredients or the manufacturing process. Most store-bought soaps are laden with synthetic fillers and additives, and though they may be labeled "pure," they are not necessarily wholesome.

Milk: The Natural Cosmetic

No one knows who first added milk to soap, though milk has been used as an ingredient in cosmetics and therapeutic treatments in different cultures for thousands of years. Centuries ago, Cleopatra indulged in luxurious milk baths to preserve her legendary beauty. The soothing and moisturizing qualities of milk have made it an increasingly popular ingredient in commercial soaps, especially over the last 30 years.

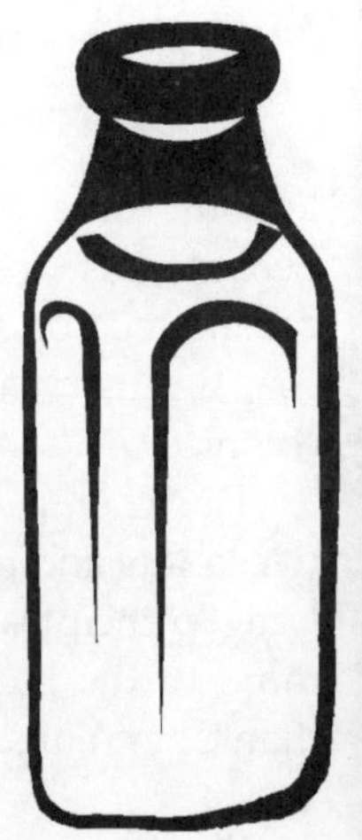

Milk is rich in proteins, vitamins, and minerals. Chemically, milk is a lipoprotein: It's made up of lipids plus protein. (A lipid is an organic substance that's insoluble in water and is usually somewhat greasy to the touch.) Lipids, found in most skin creams in the form of animal or vegetable oil or wax, help seal in moisture.

Milk is unique in its natural ability to moisturize and nourish the skin. It is a fragile miracle of nature that cannot be synthetically reproduced. But its gentle properties are easily destroyed.

Milk Is a Food

Milk is not a beverage; it is a food. It is the fluid secreted by the mammary glands of female mammals and is a complete food for the young of each species. Milk has a very high nutritional value for humans. It contains all the known and essential amino acids that we cannot synthesize in sufficient quantities.

When the term *milk* is used in North America, it is generally assumed to refer to cow's milk. In other areas of the world, however, milk may mean something different. For example, in India, buffalo milk is commonly consumed. Nomadic tribes in the Middle East drink horse milk. Goat's milk is very common in European and Middle Eastern countries, and milk from sheep is used to make excellent cheeses in Europe. Laplanders — natives of northern Sweden, Norway, Finland, or Russia — drink reindeer milk.

Animal milk has been used as a food since before recorded history. Cheese is mentioned in the Book of Job. Hindu writings dating to before 1400 B.C. refer to the use of butter as food.

Ancient Greeks, Romans, and Scythians did not use butter as food. Instead, they applied butter to skin injuries, used the soot of burned butter as an ointment for sore eyes, and considered pure butter to be an excellent hair dressing.

Not All Milk Is Created Equal

The composition of milk can vary drastically among animal species. Even within the same species, there are individual differences. Among other components, milk contains proteins, vitamins, and minerals. These individual ingredients can cause variations in soaps.

The amount of protein in both cow's and goat's milk is 3.5%. Milk has even more protein than eggs. Naturally, soap made with milk is also protein rich. This unique property makes milk-based soaps a favorite for delicate complexions.

Milk also has lots of vitamin A, which is converted from carotene by the liver. Carotene levels can fluctuate according to the lactating animal's diet. Animals that graze on lush, springtime green pastures produce milk that is higher in carotene.

Carotene affects the color of milk. Low levels cause milk to be very white, while high levels make it appear more off-white or creamy yellow. Soaps made with milk may have subtle color variations from the different levels of carotene.

Milk is an important source of minerals. In addition to calcium, milk contains potassium, sodium, magnesium, and phosphorus, plus small amounts of other minerals such as lithium and strontium.

The percentage of ash in milk reveals the amount of minerals that it contains. Milk ash is white milk that has been dried and then burned until it forms a fine, pale powder. The ash content of goat's and cow's milk is similar: Goat is 0.79% and cow is 0.73%. The ash in milk helps it to remain stable when it is combined with lye during the soapmaking process.

Cow's Milk or Goat's Milk?

Which is the best milk to use for soapmaking? The answer is—it depends. Both goat's and cow's milk make excellent milk soaps. If you live near both a cow and a goat dairy, you have the best of both worlds. If you do not have easy access to goat's milk, your choice has been made for you: Use cow's milk and don't give the question another thought.

Whole Milk, 2%, Skim, or Powdered?

In soapmaking, fat is critical to the saponifying process, so the fat content of milk is important. The standard fat content of commercial, processed cow's milk is 3%. Milk that is sold as low in fat

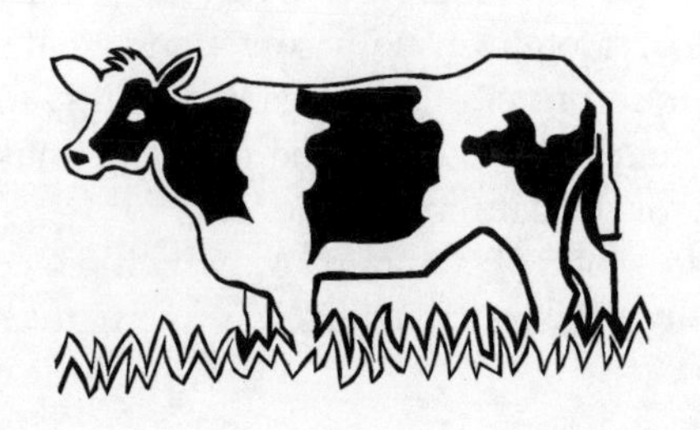

has 2% fat content, while skim has almost no fat at all. Powdered milk has nearly all of the fat removed as well. Use milk that has the highest fat content possible for the best soapmaking results. Do not be tempted to use low-fat, skim, or powdered milk: Use whole milk.

Raw or Pasteurized?

Where it is available, raw (unpasteurized) whole milk fresh from the farm has one advantage over milk from the store: Raw milk has a higher fat content than commercial milk. It is not unusual to find that the fat content of raw cow's milk exceeds 4%. Raw whole milk, if available, is the best choice, though pasteurized whole milk purchased from the grocer works fine.

Homogenized or Not?

In cow's milk, the fat globules are large and buoyant. When cow's milk is undisturbed, the fat globules rise to the top and form cream. Cow's milk is homogenized, or blended, until the fat globules are small enough to remain suspended in the milk. The fat globules in goat's milk are much smaller than those in cow's milk. A very thin cream line may occur in goat's milk that has been left undisturbed for eight or more hours, but most of the cream remains suspended in the milk, so homogenization is unnecessary. Whether or not the milk is homogenized does not affect its qualities for soapmaking, as homogenization does not change fat content.

Cream or Half-and-Half?

Whipping cream, heavy cream, and half-and-half can be used in place of whole milk in soapmaking. The resulting soap is superfatted, because of the higher fat content found in the cream-based products. When you use cream, the proportion of lye to fat is changed. In addition, not all of the fat is bound chemically during the saponification process. Using cream for milk-based soaps results in a moisturizing cleanser. When experimenting with creams, substitute an equal amount of cream for either part or all of the milk in the recipe.

Note: *In goat's milk, the fat globules are much smaller and more difficult to separate from the milk. To obtain goat's cream, you will need to use a cream separator. It's well worth the effort, however. Goat's cream makes soap extra rich.*

Making Molds

The recipes in this bulletin make approximately 8 pounds of soap, which means that if you want 4-ounce soap bars, you will be making 32 bars of soap with each batch. You need to make or buy molds to hold all that soap while it sets up.

Common soap molds include wood and even cardboard boxes lined with plastic or baker's paper. You should avoid any material that will corrode or leach color into the soap, so choose the molds carefully. Boxes should be about 14" x 20" x 2" deep, and the plastic lining should be smooth and wrinkle free.

Many companies sell premade soap molds. Candy and candle molds can be adapted to soapmaking, too, giving you a wide range of shapes and sizes for your homemade soap. But the cost of enough molds for 8 pounds of soap can be prohibitive.

Instead, try using white vinyl window expanders or PVC pipe to make molds for your milk-based soaps. (A window expander is used on the top of vinyl windows as a gap filler during window installation.) You can purchase expanders from most vinyl window manufacturers. The expanders usually come in 16' lengths with interior measurements of 1½" high x 3¼" wide. Use white window expanders, as saponifying soap can absorb colors from a mold.

Line the molds with silicone bakery paper to prevent the soap from sticking. The paper can usually be purchased at bakeries in small amounts. Although you can reuse the molds, you will need to use new paper each time you make soap.

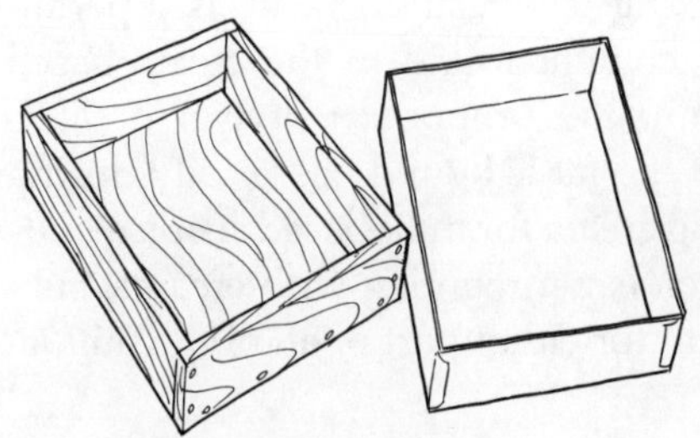

Wooden or even cardboard boxes can be used for soap molds if you line them with plastic.

BASIC MOLDS

1. Cut the expander into lengths of 69⅞ inches.

2. Seal the ends with a piece of taped PVC or vinyl, or use duct tape.

3. Cover the inside of the ends with plastic packing tape to ensure a good seal on the mold. The mold ends should be sealed inside and out.

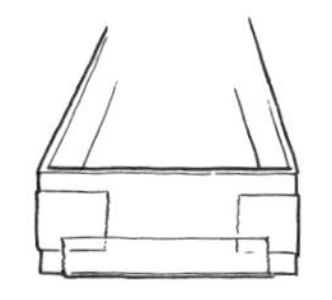

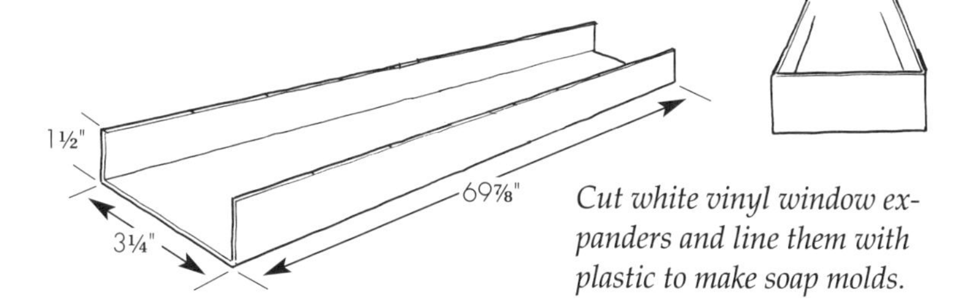

Cut white vinyl window expanders and line them with plastic to make soap molds.

4. Measure and mark the upper edge of the frame every 2¼ inches with an indelible marker. These are the cutting marks. Each mold will contain 31 bars.

5. Cut the full sheet of bakery paper into thirds.

6. Fold each third of paper so that it will fit into the mold.

7. Fit the bakery paper into the mold, smoothing out any wrinkles so that the surface of the soap will be smooth.

8. Lubricate the lined mold with spray-on corn oil. The mold is now ready for use with the recipes in this bulletin.

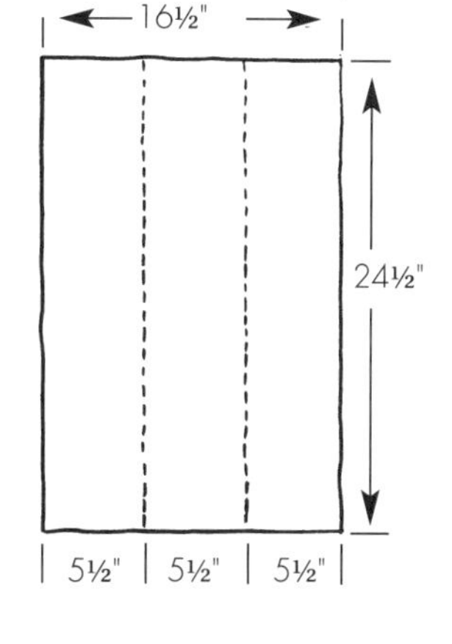

Cut the full sheet of bakery paper into thirds on the dotted lines. One sheet is enough to line one mold with overlap between sheets.

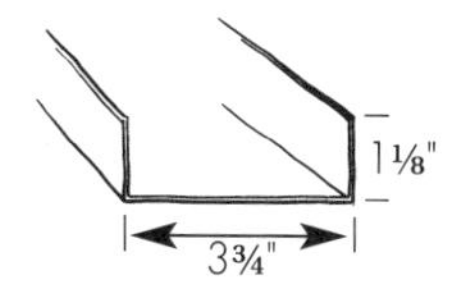

Soap Rounds

You may also want to make soap rounds. The round slices make excellent soaps that fit nicely into shaving mugs. Use a 1-foot length of round, 2-inch PVC pipe, with a removable cap on one end. You will need five or six lengths for the recipes in this bulletin. To make soap removal easier, apply liberal amounts of spray-on corn oil to the inside of the pipe. Make sure the cap is secure before pouring the liquid soap into the pipe. When the soap is hardened, remove the cap, push out the soap, and slice it into rounds.

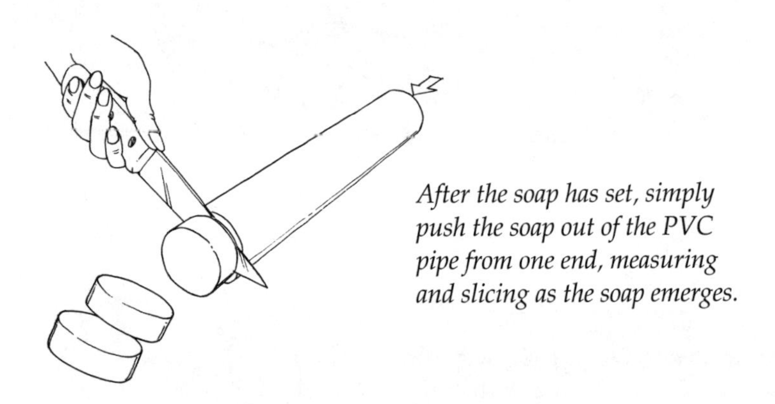

After the soap has set, simply push the soap out of the PVC pipe from one end, measuring and slicing as the soap emerges.

Working with Lye

There are a few safety precautions to follow when working with lye. Lye is a powerful and dangerous chemical that must be handled with great caution. Read this section carefully before you make soap.

You can purchase sodium hydroxide, or lye, in your grocery store in 12-ounce (340-g) containers. This is the amount needed for recipes in this bulletin and it's convenient to have the lye premeasured in a disposable container.

Lye cannot be handled with bare hands, and its fumes must not be inhaled. Lye is harmful or fatal if swallowed. Until the fat/lye mixture fully saponifies into soap (approximately 48 hours after being poured into the mold), it will burn the skin on contact.

Occasionally, the soap mixture separates after the liquid has been poured into the mold. If this happens, you must discard the batch of soap. You might be tempted to pour the batch back into the saucepan and reheat it to encourage saponification. This will not work and is extremely dangerous.

The liquid is highly corrosive and lye is very sensitive to being heated. The goal of soapmaking is to temper lye's hot nature. If you heat it, you can cause the lye to become chemically aggressive and lose control over the process. Never reheat the mixture.

Follow these safe practices when working with lye:

- Read and follow the precautionary statements on the lye container.
- Make sure the product you purchase contains only sodium hydroxide. Read the label carefully; some brands contain additives that will interfere with the saponification process.
- Always wear safety glasses. Don't risk exposing your eyes to the lye.
- Always wear rubber gloves. If you spill any lye on your skin, immediately wash the affected area in cold water.

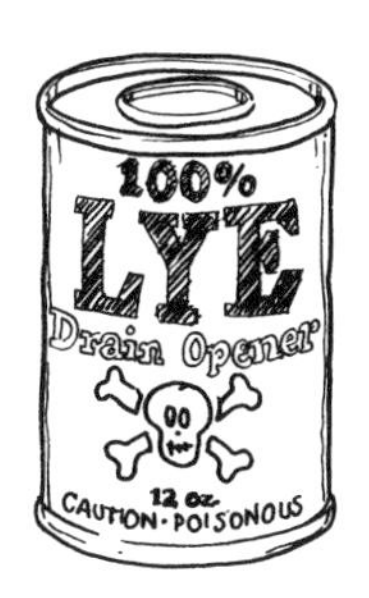

- Work in a well-ventilated room, near an open window if possible. Do not inhale the fumes. Leave the room immediately for a few minutes when the milk and lye are first mixed if the fumes become too strong.
- Thoroughly clean every utensil, container, counter, and tabletop that was used for soapmaking immediately after the soap is poured into the molds.

Tips for a Safe Work Environment

There are important precautions that you should take before soapmaking can safely begin. The process will take your undivided attention from start to finish, so allow yourself plenty of time free from distractions, phone calls, and other interruptions.

- *Work on a stable surface.* The work surface should be a roomy, stable area such as a cleared kitchen countertop. Avoid rickety tables.
- *Cover the work surface.* Cover all work surfaces with newspaper or plastic to protect them from accidental splashes or spills.

- *Lay out the equipment.* Lay out and organize the soapmaking equipment so it is easily accessible. Once you start to mix the ingredients, it will be too late to look for equipment.
- *Dedicate the equipment to soapmaking.* Soapmaking equipment is laboratory equipment. It should be used only for soapmaking. Never use it for cooking once it's been used to make soap.
- *Start with new equipment.* Foodstuffs can ruin a batch of soap. It's best to invest in new soapmaking equipment. You can find everything you need at a kitchen supply store or a supermarket.
- *Do not allow children to help.* Young children should be supervised away from the soapmaking work area. Older children may observe from a safe distance, though they should leave the room when the milk and lye are first mixed because of the fumes. Rubber gloves and safety glasses are a must for their protection — even if they are not helping in the process.

Before You Make the First Batch

Soapmaking is a process that cannot be hurried. This is especially true with milk soap. Every batch will be slightly different, even if you follow the recipe exactly every time. Allow for each batch to develop its individual character in its own time. Keep the following points in mind before you make your first batch:

- *Soapmaking is a lengthy process.* At first, it will take you several hours to make a batch of soap. Because the batch must be continually stirred while portions are blended, it's much easier to work with another person.
- *Take careful notes.* If you document every detail of each batch, right down to the weather, you'll create a running record that will tell you what works best.
- *Choose quality ingredients.* Do not lessen the quality of your soap by cutting corners to save a few pennies. Soap that is not as lathery, long lasting, nice smelling, or as even colored as it should be will waste the time and money you have invested.

- *Measure accurately.* Soapmaking is a science. For best results, measure as precisely as possible. This means measuring by weight, not volume. A good digital scale will give you accurate control and your records will be more detailed and dependable.
- *Be patient.* Once the soap is poured into molds, it must be allowed to sit for 24 – 48 hours until it is hard enough to be cut. Then, bars must be allowed to cure, undisturbed, for six weeks.

Preparing the Milk

You'll need to prepare the milk at least two days before you make the soap, as it must be frozen and then thawed before use. Freezing milk increases its stability, making it more effective in the soapmaking process.

In addition, milk must be pasteurized before it can be used as an ingredient in soap. Commercially sold milk is already pasteurized. Raw milk purchased fresh from a farm and goat's milk have not been pasteurized.

To pasteurize milk, slowly heat it to 155°F (68°C), measuring with a glass candy thermometer. Hold the milk at this temperature for 1 minute, then cover the pan and allow the milk to cool.

Once the milk has cooled, pour it into a freezer-safe container (don't use glass), leaving room for expansion. Allow the milk to freeze solid. The milk can be stored in the freezer for several months. Remove the milk from the freezer and thaw the day before you're ready to make soap. Once it has thawed, the milk is ready to use.

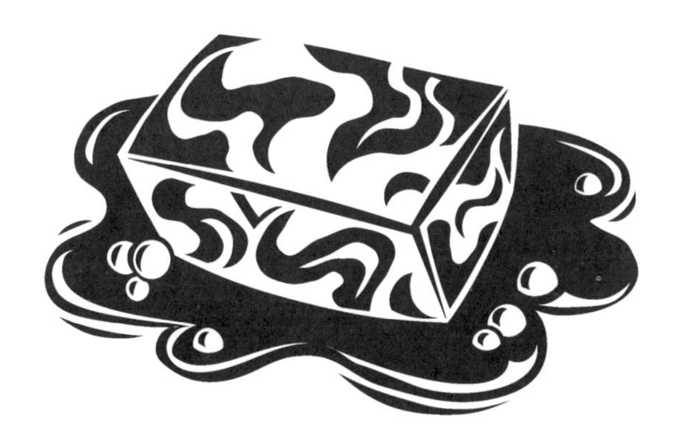

Basic Equipment

Many of the tools you'll need to make soap are probably already in your kitchen. Remember to use the soapmaking equipment for soapmaking only. You will need:

- Plastic wrap and newspaper to cover work surfaces
- Two 8-quart (7.5-l) stainless-steel saucepans **Note:** *Never use aluminum containers or your containers and soap will be ruined.*
- Digital scale
- 4-quart (3.7-l) stainless-steel saucepan
- Ice-water bath: Fill the sink with cold water, then add 4–6 trays of ice cubes
- Several 8-ounce plastic cups
- 16-ounce (454-g) glass measuring cup
- 2 heavy-duty plastic or stainless-steel spoons **Note:** *Never use wooden spoons; the lye will destroy the wood fibers.*
- Glass candy thermometer
- Plastic ladle
- Blender
- Plastic spatula
- Narrow-blade putty knife
- Trisquare
- Molds
- Curing rack

Note: *Large plastic bread racks work well as curing racks. Don't use wood, aluminum, or steel curing racks, as these materials react with the soap while it is curing, ruining both the rack and the soap.*

Let's Make Soap!

Understand the safety precautions of working with lye. Caustic soda is very dangerous and can cause serious burns. Carefully read and follow the safety instructions each time you make soap.

The first time you make a basic, milk-based soap, you can expect the process to take about 3 hours. After you become more experienced, you'll need about 1½ hours, including cleanup and barring any unforeseen chemical complications. Before you begin, review the list and set aside the ingredients and equipment. Reread the safety precautions for working with lye.

Cover all work surfaces with plastic or newspaper. Lay out your soapmaking equipment so it is within reach, including the molds. Wear gloves and safety glasses at all times.

Well-made milk soap is created with the maximum amount of milk that can be included in proportion to the lye and fat used in each batch. There has to be a substantial amount of milk in every batch to react properly with the lye. Ideally, each 4-ounce bar of soap should have 1½ – 2 ounces of its weight in milk.

Fine cosmetic soaps are often made with a combination of liquid vegetable oils and vegetable shortening. Vegetable shortening usually comes from soybeans. It is economical and readily available at grocery stores and makes an excellent milk-based soap. Olive oil is a good moisturizer. Using extra-light olive oil reduces its slight odor and makes a lighter-colored soap. Safflower and canola oils add foaming action to soap, helping to create the luxurious lathers associated with good soap.

The biggest challenge in making milk-based soap is adding the lye to 6 cups of milk. It can be tricky to combine the caustic chemical with such a large volume of milk. For best results, practice making several batches of soap using the basic recipe before making soap with added ingredients.

You'll need help at several points during the process. Working with a partner makes the soapmaking experience much easier and more enjoyable.

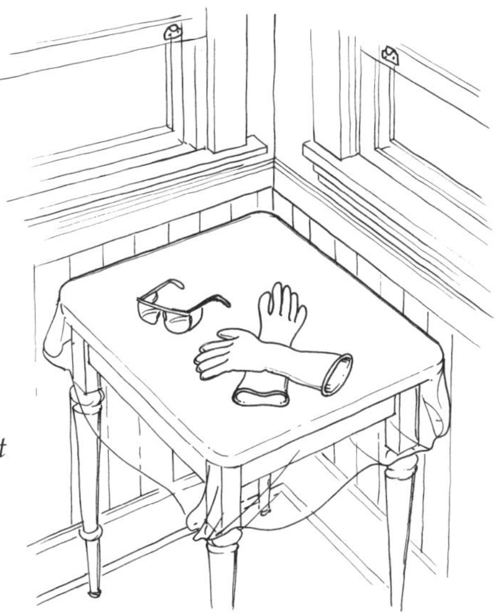

A safe and stable work area and good safety equipment are the most important factors in successful soapmaking.

BASIC MILK-BASED SOAP RECIPE

- **3 pounds (1.36 kg) pure vegetable shortening**
- **17 ounces (482 g) extra-light olive oil**
- **12 ounces (341 g) safflower oil**
- **8 ounces (227 g) canola oil**
- **3 pounds (1.36 kg, or approximately 6 cups) cold milk, prepared for soapmaking**
- **12 ounces (312 g) pure lye (sodium hydroxide)**
- **1 ounce (28.4 g) borax**
- **½ ounce (7.1 g) white sugar**
- **½ ounce (7.1 g) glycerin**

YIELD: 32 (4-OUNCE) BARS

Prepare the Fats and Milk

1. Melt the vegetable shortening in an 8-quart saucepan over low heat.

2. Add the liquid oils to the shortening. Heat the combined ingredients just until the shortening is completely melted, then immediately remove from the heat. Take care not to overheat or scorch the oils, or you will ruin them for soapmaking. Set aside the oil mixture until you are ready to add the lye/milk mixture.

3. Create an ice-water bath by filling the sink with cold water and adding 4–6 trays of ice cubes to the water.

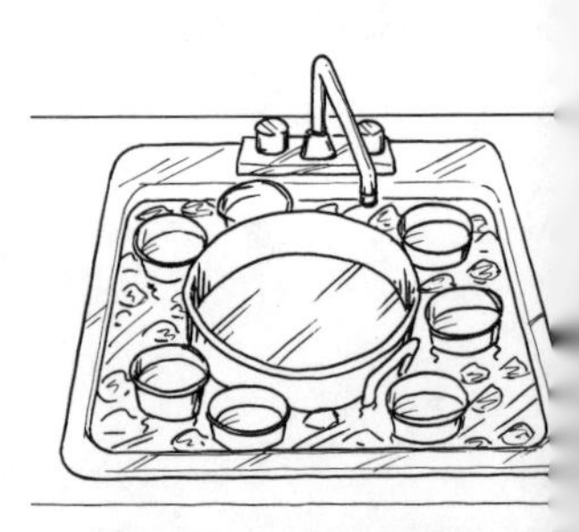

4. Place the prepared, cold milk into a 4-quart stainless-steel saucepan. Carefully place the saucepan in the ice water.

5. Place several plastic cups filled with water around the floating pan to stabilize it.

Add the Lye to the Milk

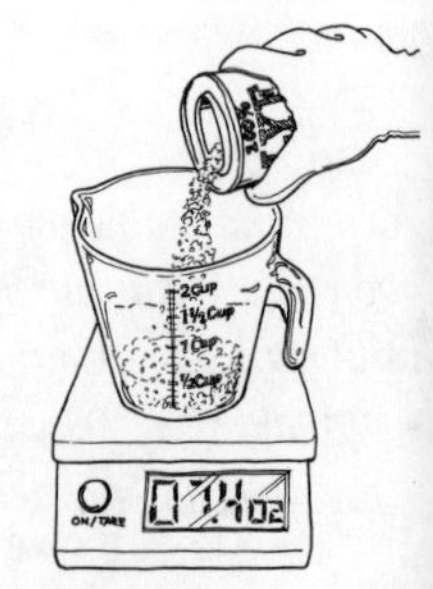

1. Wearing safety glasses and gloves, measure the lye into a 16-ounce glass measuring cup, using a digital scale for accuracy.

2. Very slowly pour the lye into the cold milk in the ice-water bath, stirring constantly with a heavy-duty plastic or stainless-steel spoon.

Caution: *This pouring process should take no less than 15 minutes. It's very important to introduce the lye slowly into the milk so that the lye does not reach extreme temperatures and react with the milk, causing the milk to burn.*

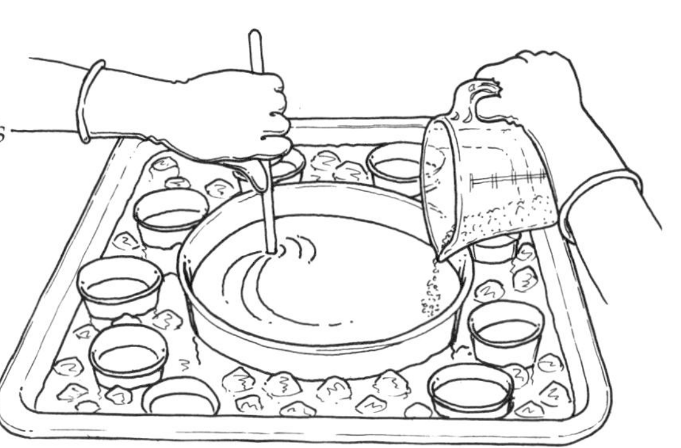

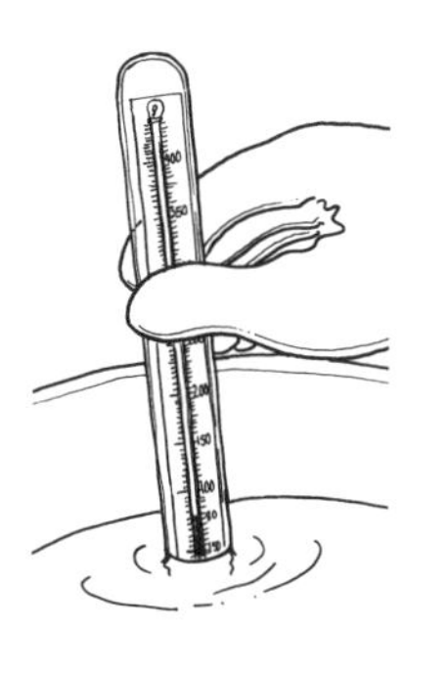

3. Use a candy thermometer to monitor the temperature of the lye/milk mixture constantly, taking care not to let the temperature fall below 80°F (27°C). You want to keep the mixture cool enough to prevent the milk from scorching, but warm enough to prevent the milk and lye from saponifying. Saponification occurs between the milk and the lye at this temperature because there is enough fat in the milk to cause this action. The two main mistakes you might make at this point are allowing the lye/milk mixture to get too cool and letting it sit too long before combining it with the oils. Both of these scenarios could cause the mixture to congeal into a noxious and useless custard-textured mass that would need to be scooped out of the pan instead of poured. So guard the temperature and keep stirring. Keep the temperature of the mixture right at 80°F, and remove the lye/milk mixture from the ice-water bath as soon as the lye and milk are combined. You will notice that the milk turns a bright yellow once the lye has been successfully combined with the milk.

Combine All Ingredients

1. Over low heat, reheat the oils to a temperature of 125°F (52°C), taking care not to scorch the oils. Remove from the heat.

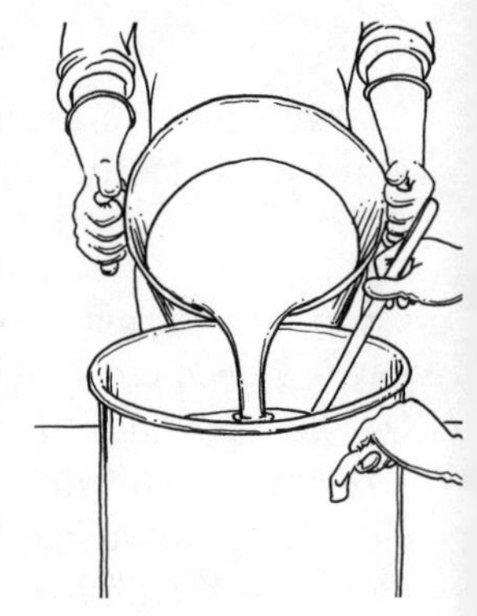

2. Slowly pour the lye/milk mixture into the oils.

3. Add the borax, sugar, and glycerin. Stir the mixture constantly, taking care not to splash any. The mixture will begin to warm as the lye reacts. You might also notice that the mixture doesn't want to combine and that it separates readily if you stop stirring. Just be patient.

Blend the Soap Mixture

1. Using a plastic ladle, scoop evenly mixed amounts of the soap mixture into the blender. Fill the blender halfway.

Caution: *Secure the lid on the blender carefully before turning it on!*

2. Run the blender for 1 minute on medium speed, remembering to keep stirring the remaining soap mixture at the same time. The liquid in the blender will turn a pale cream color.

3. After 1 minute, pour the contents of the blender into the second 8-quart saucepan. This is where having a partner is critical — you now have two saucepans to stir and the blender to operate.

4. Repeat steps 1–3 until all of the original mixture of oils and lye/milk has been blended.

5. Quickly wash out the first saucepan and dry thoroughly.

6. Now do the same thing all over again, transferring from the full saucepan to the blender for 1 minute, and then into the now empty saucepan.

7. After the second blending, the liquid is ready to pour

into molds. You should see little or no separation of the oils from the rest of the mixture. After the second blending, the mixture should have thickened up somewhat, but even if it seems a little thin, it will still be ready for the molds. If it really seems too thin, you can blend it a third time.

Pour the Soap into the Molds

1. Pour the mixture into the prepared mold(s). To prevent the soap from seeping through the bakery-paper liner, use a spatula to press down on the liner until the soap flows over the liner and weighs it down.

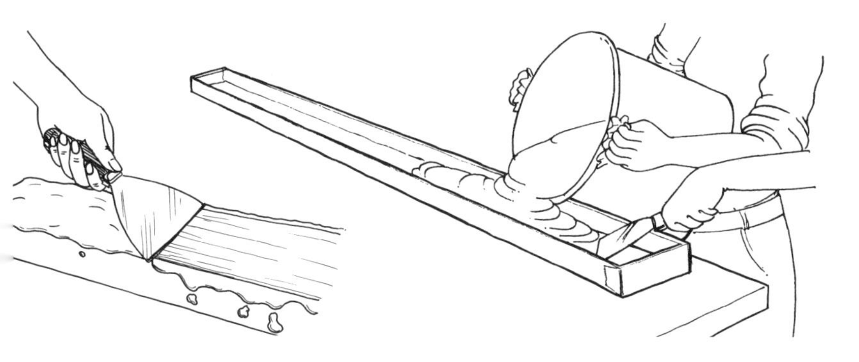

2. Once a mold is full, you can screed the surface with the spatula to smooth out the surface of the soap: Slowly pull the flat edge of the spatula across the entire surface of the mold, from one end to the other.

3. Allow the saponifying liquid to sit uncovered and undisturbed in a draft-free area. After 12 hours, you may notice sweatlike beads of moisture on the surface of the soap. These usually evaporate, but if they don't, you can gently wipe them off with a paper towel before cutting the bars.

4. After 24 hours, use the narrow-blade putty knife to cut the bars. Set the trisquare parallel to each 2¼-inch mark to guide a straight cut. Then slice each bar straight down with the putty knife, sliding it from one side of the mold to the other. Do not wait more than 24 hours to cut, or the soap will become too brittle.

5. Cut the entire strip of bars, then remove one bar to check its hardness. If the bar holds its shape, remove all the bars and place them on the curing rack. If the soap does not hold its shape, allow it to remain in the mold for another 24 hours. Check it every 4 hours until it is ready.

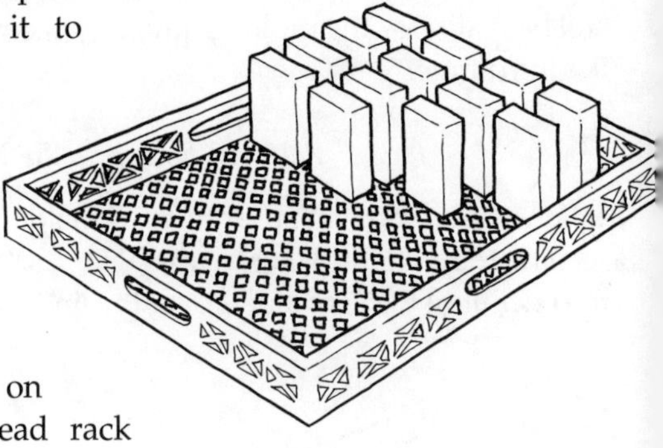

6. As soon as the bars are ready, place them on the curing rack. If you stand the soap bars on the narrow ends, a bread rack measuring 26½" x 22" will hold three batches of soap, or 96 bars.

7. Allow the bars to cure for six weeks in a dry, cool room. Cover lightly with plastic wrap to protect the bars from dust.

Failure to Saponify

It happens to the best of soapmakers once in a while — a batch of soap refuses to saponify. When you hit a stubborn batch that refuses to set up, starting over is the best solution. If the mixture becomes overheated, the milk will not mix with the lye. The milk will change from an orange color to a burnt orange and float to the top of the mixture. There is no alternative but to dispose of the batch and start over.

Another problem might occur when the lye/milk mixture cools too long before being combined with the oils. The mixture will become custardlike and will have to be scooped out of the pan. You can still add it to the oils, though. Usually the blender will mix it well enough so that it poses no further problems. The lye/milk mixture will be easier to work with if you maintain the temperature so it can be poured out of the pan.

Occasionally the soap separates after it has been poured into the molds. The mixture will not saponify. Again, the only solution is to discard the batch and start over.

Loofah Sponge Soap Scrubs

These sponge scrubs are useful for showering and also make great gifts. They are a nice alternative to molded soaps as well, as they need no other container.

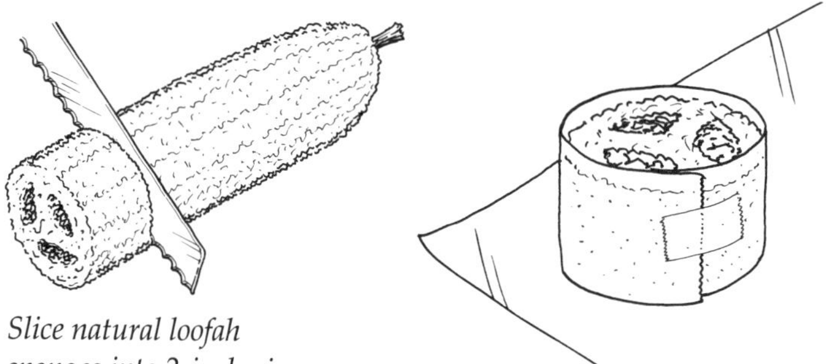

Slice natural loofah sponges into 2-inch pieces.

Wrap the outside of each loofah piece in waxed paper and set the pieces on end on another piece of waxed paper.

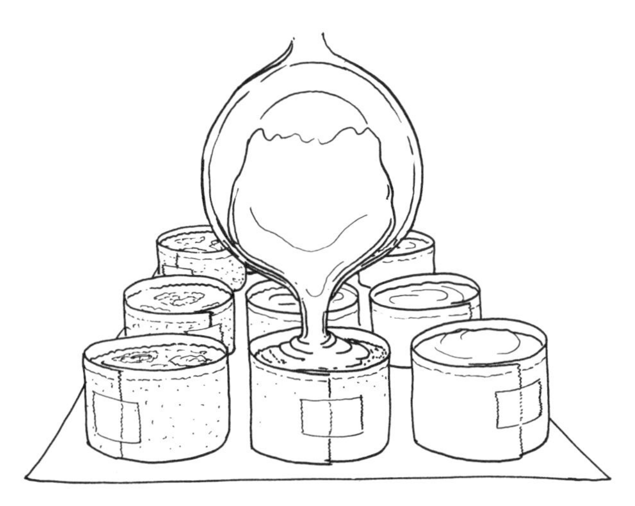

Fill the hollow insides with liquid soap. Allow the soap-filled loofahs to cure for six weeks.

Additional Soap Ingredients

Once you've gotten the knack of making basic milk soap, there are many natural ingredients you can add. Use your imagination when adding ingredients.

Herbs

Herbs, fresh or dried, are a wonderful addition to milk-based soap. Lavender, chamomile, and rosemary add a distinct identity to the soap, as do rose petals. Herbs will not keep their original color; most fade in reaction to the lye. The aromas and textures are captured, though.

Exfoliants

A number of ingredients add exfoliating qualities to soap, gently scraping away dead skin cells and allowing new cells to breathe.

Oatmeal. Oatmeal soap has been an enduring favorite for generations. The addition of ground oatmeal to soap gives it a rich texture that is suitable for normal, oily, and dry skin types. Soap containing oatmeal has a lovely ivory/tan color.

Cornmeal. Cornmeal soap has a strong but not harsh cleansing property that makes it a perfect all-purpose soap. It has a golden yellow color and a pleasant, naturally sweet fragrance.

Bran. In addition to its mild exfoliating qualities, bran soap is a lovely pale ivory in color with brown specks of bran throughout.

Almond meal. Ground almonds help create a gentle cleansing bar that exfoliates and moisturizes dry skin types.

Eggshells. This surprising ingredient has powerful cleansing abilities and is suitable for hand soaps. Its abrasiveness is too harsh for a facial bar, however.

Moisturizers

Cocoa butter. This is the pure cocoa fat extracted from ground and crushed cocoa beans. Cocoa butter is considered to be nourishing as well as moisturizing for the skin.

Lanolin. Lanolin is the grease or fat that comes from sheep's wool. It is used in cosmetics as a neutral, non-irritating base for ointments and creams because of its excellent moisturizing qualities. Sheep shearers rarely suffer from dry, chapped hands. Lanolin is very thick and tacky and has a dark yellowish color with a strong odor. Once the soap is made, however, the odor disappears. Use only nonhydrous lanolin for soapmaking. (Nonhydrous lanolin has never had water or other ingredients whipped into it to make it creamy.) Your pharmacist will carry it in 1-pound (454-g) quantities.

Healing Ingredients

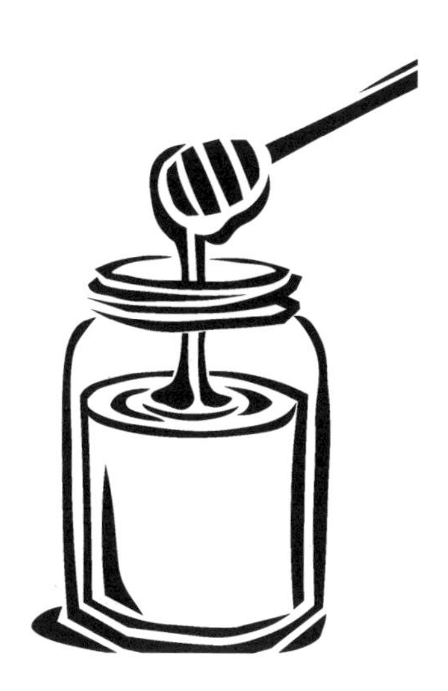

Aloe vera. Famous for its healing qualities, the gel-like substance from the aloe vera plant produces a mild, all-purpose soap that is soothing to the skin.

Honey. Honey is a soothing ingredient for soaps. It's a source of vitamins, minerals, and amino acids and has slight antiseptic properties. It's an especially good ingredient for delicate skin.

Colors from Nature

Natural, milk-based soaps will range from the pale green of rosemary soap to a light brown if you use cinnamon and cloves, and from pale yellow from cornmeal to varying shades of creams and tans from other ingredients. Because of its caustic nature, you won't see the strong colors that are found in store-bought soaps. Adding chopped herbs, plant materials, or ground grains will provide a pretty speckled look and a bit more texture to the soap.

Selecting a Scent

As with natural colors, many natural scents are destroyed during saponification. Synthetic perfumes and colors offer a wide array of choices, but lack the character and goodness of natural products.

Fragrances and colors from natural ingredients often go hand in hand. For example, adding cornmeal makes the soap golden yellow with a sweet corn smell. Cinnamon produces a brownish soap that smells like that spice.

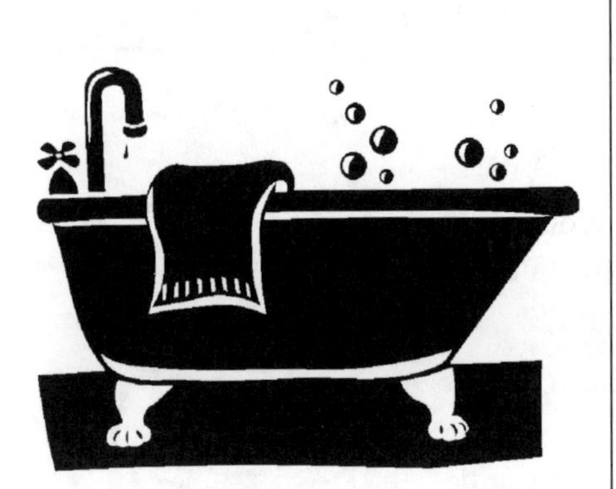

Soap Scents

The following are strong enough to withstand the saponification process.

Almond	Orange
Cinnamon	Patchouli
Citronella	Peach
Cloves	Pennyroyal
Eucalyptus	Peppermint
Jasmine	Rose
Lavender	Rosemary
Lemon	Sage
Musk	Vanilla

Essential Oils or Fragrance Oils?

Essential oils are highly concentrated extracts derived from the leaves, berries, flower, petals, twigs, bark, or stems of plants through distillation or expression. The oils usually bear the scent or fragrance of the original plant. Essential oils are also believed to have therapeutic properties. Prices for essential oils vary and can be quite high, depending on the plant type. But a little goes a long way.

Fragrance oils are synthetically produced imitations of plant essences. They are far less expensive than essential oils and are less vulnerable to spoilage.

Specialty Recipes

Now that you've made several batches of soap, you can start experimenting with other ingredients. All of the following recipes make 32 four-ounce bars.

Complexion Soaps

Use these soaps for caring for different types of complexions.

HONEY CREAM SOAP

This soap is especially mild and good for delicate skin. The goat's cream makes the soap extra rich. If you can't obtain goat's cream, substitute cow's cream.

Follow the procedure for making soap, but with these substitutions:

¼ **ounce (7.1 g) honey in place of the sugar**

In place of the 3 pounds of prepared milk, use:

1 **pound (454 g or approximately 2 cups) prepared goat or cow's cream, plus**

2 **pounds (908 g or approximately 4 cups) prepared cow's milk**

Special instructions:
Add the cream to the milk before combining the milk with the oils.

OATMEAL SOAP

Oatmeal soap is excellent for oily complexions. The coarse oatmeal is a good exfoliant. This recipe is scented with fragrant vanilla and almond oils.

Follow the procedure for making soap, adding these ingredients to the recipe:

½ **cup (118 ml) rolled oats**

¼ **ounce (7.1 g) almond fragrance oil**

¼ **ounce (7.1 g) vanilla fragrance oil**

Special instructions:
Blend the rolled oats for 60 seconds or until you get a medium-coarse powder. Add the refined oatmeal to the liquid when it's blended for the first time. Add the almond and vanilla oils to the liquid when it's blended for the second time.

ALMOND JOY

Sweet almond oil, ground almonds, and almond fragrance create a wonderful soap that works well for dry skin.

Follow the procedure for making soap, but with this substitution:

20 ounces (568 g) sweet almond oil for the safflower and canola oils

Also add the following ingredients to the recipe:

½ cup (118 m) raw almonds
½ ounce (14.2 g) almond fragrance oil

Special instructions:
Combine the almond oil with the other oils at the beginning of the process. Blend the raw almonds for 60 seconds or until you get a coarse powder. Add the almond meal to the liquid when it's blended for the first time. Then add the almond oil to the liquid when it's blended for the second time.

Scented Soaps

These soaps are reminiscent of country gardens.

PEACHES AND CREAM

This creamy soap has a wonderful peachy scent. Goat's cream makes the soap rich and creamy. If goat's cream is unavailable, substitute cow's cream.

In place of the 3 pounds of prepared milk, use:

1 pound (454 g or approximately 2 cups) prepared goat's or cow's cream, plus
2 pounds (908 g or approximately 4 cups) prepared cow's milk

Also add the following ingredient to the recipe:

½ ounce (14.2 g) peach fragrance oil

Special instructions:
Add the cream to the milk before combining the milk with the oils.

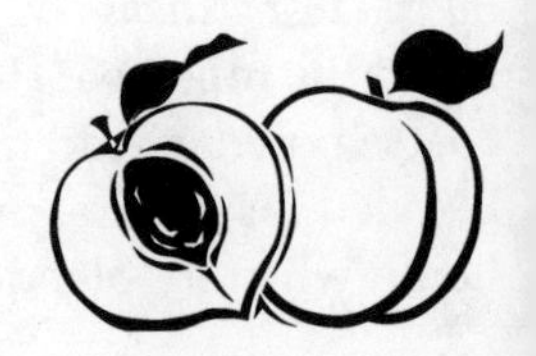

ROMANTIC ROSE

Delicate petals and the enchanting fragrance of roses enhance this romantic soap.

Follow the procedure for making soap, but with these substitutions:

- **11 ounces (312 g) safflower oil rather than 12 ounces (341 g)**
- **9 ounces (170 g) canola oil rather than 8 ounces (227 g)**

Also add the following ingredients to the recipe:

- **¾ cup (177 ml) dried or fresh red rose petals**
- **½ ounce (14.2 g) rose fragrance oil**

Special instructions:
Add the rose petals and rose oil to the liquid when it's blended for the second time.

LAVENDER LACE

Lavender is a timeless fragrance, with a scent that evokes a gentler era and enduring innocence.

Follow the procedure for making soap, but with this substitution:

- **7 ounces (199 g) canola oil rather than 8 ounces (227 g)**

Also add the following ingredients to the recipe:

- **¾ cup (177 ml) dried lavender flowers**
- **50 drops lavender essential oil**

Special instructions:
Add the lavender flowers to the liquid when it's blended for the first time. Add the lavender oil to the liquid when it's blended for the second time.

ROSEMARY MIST

This earthy soap has a lovely pale green color and the stimulating scent of rosemary.

Follow the procedure for making soap, but with these substitutions:

10 ounces (284 g) safflower oil rather than 12 ounces (341 g)

7 ounces (199 g) canola oil rather than 8 ounces (227 g)

Also add the following ingredients to the recipe:

⅓ cup (79 ml) dried rosemary

½ ounce (14.2 g) rosemary essential oil

Special instructions:
Blend the rosemary for 60 seconds or until you get a coarse powder. Add the blended rosemary to the liquid when it's blended for the first time. Add the rosemary oil to the liquid when it's blended for the second time.

Moisturizing Soaps

Natural moisturizers help keep skin feeling smooth.

SHEPHERD'S PRIDE

This soap contains pure lanolin and aloe vera, both renowned for their healing and moisturizing properties. Scented with jasmine, this soap is excellent for dry skin.

Follow the procedure for making soap, but with this substitution:

4 ounces (113 g) canola oil rather than 8 ounces (227 g)

Also add the following ingredients to the recipe:

4 ounces (113 g) lanolin

½ ounce (14.2 g) aloe vera

½ ounce (14.2 g) jasmine fragrance oil

Special instructions:
Melt the lanolin with the other oils. Add the aloe vera and jasmine oil to the liquid when it's blended for the second time.

COCOA BUTTER SOAP

The tropical richness of cocoa butter blends with coconut and almond fragrances to create a rich bath bar that is nourishing to your skin and senses.

Follow the procedure for making soap, but with these substitutions:

10 ounces (284 g) safflower oil rather than 12 ounces (341 g)

6 ounces (170 g) canola oil rather than 8 ounces (227 g)

Also add the following ingredients to the recipe:

4 ounces (113 g) cocoa butter

½ ounce (14.2 g) almond fragrance oil

½ ounce (14.2 g) coconut fragrance oil

Special instructions:
Melt the cocoa butter with the other oils. Add the almond oil to the liquid when it's blended for the second time.

Scrubbing Soaps

These soaps use natural additives as exfoliants.

CORNMEAL SCRUB

Add cornmeal to create a gently abrasive soap. Its golden color and fresh citrus smell make this a favorite soap to keep in the laundry or at the kitchen sink for quick scrubs.

Follow the procedure for making soap, but with this substitution:

10 ounces (284 g) safflower oil rather than 12 ounces (341 g)

Also add the following ingredients to the recipe:

½ cup (118 ml) yellow cornmeal

¼ ounce (7.1 g) orange essential oil

¼ ounce lemon essential oil

Special instructions:
Add the cornmeal to the liquid when it's blended for the first time. Add the orange and lemon oils to the liquid when it's blended for the second time.

NITTY-GRITTY SOAP

Nothing cleans hardworking hands better than this super scrub soap made with ground eggshells. When the liquid soap is poured into the mold, the eggshells will sink to the bottom, making the finished bar smooth on one side and abrasive on the other. Cedar adds a nice fragrance to this extra-powerful scrubbing soap.

Follow the procedure for making soap, but with this substitution:

7 ounces (199 g) canola oil rather than 8 ounces (227 g)

Also add the following ingredients to the recipe:

¼ cup (59 ml) finely ground eggshells (approximately 1 dozen dried shells)

50 drops cedar essential oil

Special instructions:
Blend the dried eggshells to a fine powder. Add the cedar oil to the liquid when it's blended for the second time.

HAPPY CAMPER

Folks who enjoy the outdoors will really appreciate this soap. It contains citronella and eucalyptus oils to keep the bugs at bay — naturally.

Follow the procedure for making soap, but with these substitutions:

10 ounces (284 g) safflower oil rather than 12 ounces (341 g)

7 ounces (199 g) canola oil rather than 8 ounces (227 g)

Also add the following ingredients to the recipe:

½ ounce (14.2 g) citronella essential oil

½ ounce (14.2 g) eucalyptus essential oil

Special instructions:
Add the citronella and eucalyptus oils to the liquid when it's blended for the second time.

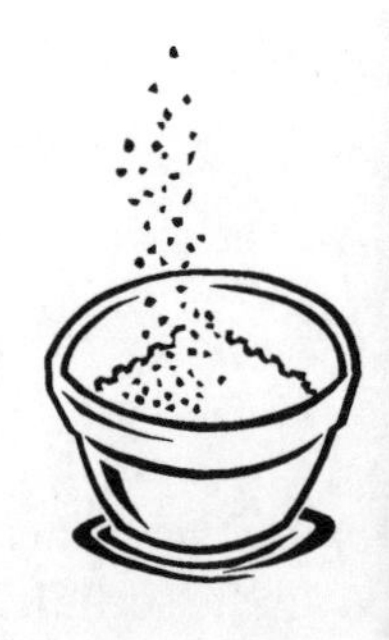

Preserving Milk-Based Soaps

Generally, homemade soap does not need preservatives to protect it from becoming stale or rancid. As it ages, all soap becomes more effective. Correctly made, the soap recipes in this bulletin have no time limit on the curing process. You do not need to worry about increasing the shelf life of the soap.

Packaging the Final Product

Homemade soap makes a wonderful, useful, and unusual gift. Beautiful and gentle milk-based soap is a gift the lucky recipient will remember long after the bar is used up.

Good packaging reflects the quality of your product. You will want your package to convey the charm and uniqueness that cannot be found in commercially purchased soap.

Be creative in your packaging. Try a few of these ideas, or come up with your own:

- Wrap the soap in calico fabric and tie it with a satin ribbon.
- Roll up a solid-colored washcloth or hand towel and tie a fabric-wrapped bar of soap to it with raffia.
- Fold a pretty kitchen washcloth and tie an unwrapped bar of soap to it with a long piece of raffia. With a hot-glue gun, glue a star anise in the center of the bow.
- Purchase pretty country mugs, then put about 1 inch (2.5 cm) of fine curled wood shavings (sometimes sold as excelsior) in the bottom. Place a bar of soap in the mug and tie a raffia bow to the handle.
- Put a bar of soap in a small, brown paper bag, fold the top, punch a hole in the bag, and tie with raffia.
- Make small wooden crates that will hold two bars of soap snugly and tie them with raffia.
- Make some wooden soap dishes and tie a bar of soap onto each one.
- Purchase inexpensive baskets, put 1 inch (2.5 cm) of fine colored wood shavings in the bottom, and place two or three soaps in each.
- Purchase handmade paper, wrap bars, and add your own handmade label.

Related Titles of Interest from Storey Books

Milk-Based Soaps by Casey Makela
Soapmakers know that moisturizing milk-based soaps can be tricky to make. Now Casey Makela has developed a specialized yet simple technique for making this sought-after soap. Crafters will learn how to make classic beauty and specialty soaps. They will also learn how to turn this hobby into a money-maker! 112 pages ISBN 0-88266-984-2

The Essential Oils Book by Colleen K. Dodt
A rich resource on the many applications of aromatherapy and its uses in everyday life including aromas for the home, scents for business environments, and essences for the elderly. 160 pages ISBN 0-88266-913-3

Gifts for Herb Lovers by Betty Oppenheimer
Herb lovers can create herbal body creams, herb-printed note cards, herbal vinegar, an herb drying rack, and much more. 128 pages ISBN 0-88266-983-4

The Natural Soap Book by Susan Miller Cavitch
An inspiring exploration of the goodness of soap without chemical additives and synthetic ingredients. 192 pages ISBN 0-88266-888-9

Perfumes, Splashes & Colognes by Nancy M. Booth
With Nancy Booth's easy instructions and "Personal Scent Profile Quiz," readers will learn how to create customized perfume blends and re-create favorite commercial perfumes at a fraction of their retail price. 176 pages ISBN 0-88266-985-0

The Soapmaker's Companion by Susan Miller Cavitch
The most authoritative guide to making natural, vegetable-based soaps ever written. In addition to basic soapmaking instruction, readers will learn how to use specialty techniques like marbling, layering, and making transparent, liquid, and imprinted soaps. 288 pages ISBN 0-88266-965-6